THE RECESSION

Kama Sutra

THE RECESSION KAMA SUTRA

Summersdale Publishers Ltd
46 West Street
Chichester
West Sussex
PO19 1RP
UK

www.summersdale.com

Printed and bound in the UK by CPI Group (UK) Ltd, Croydon, CR0 4YY

ISBN: 978-1-84953-317-1

Substantial discounts on bulk quantities of Summersdale books are available to corporations, professional associations and other organisations. For details telephone Summersdale Publishers on (+44-1243-771107), fax (+44-1243-786300) or email (nicky@summersdale.com).

THE RECESSION

Kama Sutra

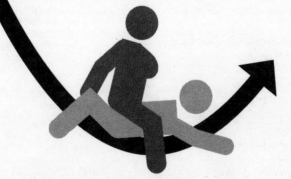

 Sarah Herman

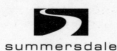

summersdale

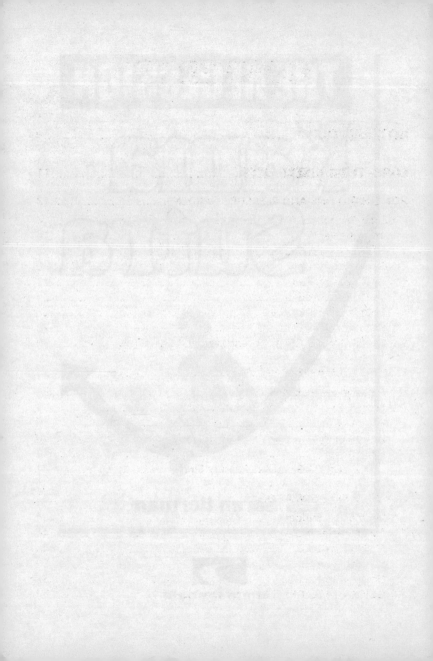

CONTENTS

INTRODUCTION

Like a sex-life dry spell that just won't end, the recession ain't going away anytime soon. If you're not getting any in the bedroom, people will tell you, 'Get out there, live your life and sex will find you!' or 'Buy a new sex toy', and my advice for making it through the recession is pretty much the same – but if you are going to buy a sex toy, make sure it's in the sale. Piles of money aren't going to suddenly appear, so it's time to do all the things you normally did, and most of the things you want, with a frisky and frugal mind. You might not be getting paid more, but this way you'll definitely be getting laid more.

While many mistakenly believe the original Kama Sutra to be an ancient Hindu sex manual, the sacred text is a more holistic guide to living that details the nature of love, family life and other pleasurable facets of the human experience. Don't worry, this book is mainly about sex (phew!), but by finding truly pleasurable and thrifty ways to be happy with less, especially if they result in your legs ending up somewhere behind your head, your whole life will feel hotter, hornier and more affordable. And remember, the more time you spend enjoying each other's rear ends, the less time you'll have to stress about making ends meet.

Those wise, bearded people said, the best things in life are free (and we all know they're talking about sex here), so why waste money on a lavish lifestyle that will dig you

into a giant hole of debt, when all you really want to do is
have someone explore your holes with their giant spade,
for free or go on a crevice-explorer adventure of your own?
Embrace a world of cheaper home improvements, fashion
fixes, daily commutes, workout regimes and more that all
lead to toe-curling orgasms and a vibrant, varied sex life.

Most of this book targets those of you who are in a romp-tastic
relationship or already have a bonking buddy you can sign up
for cash-saving copulation. But fear not sexy singletons. There
are loads of activities you can do without a partner, try out with
friends, or introduce into the workplace. That's right, not even
that hot guy/girl in accounting can escape from your quest to
cut costs and care for your sex drive. The activities are suitable
for boys and girls (of the appropriate age) of same-sex and
heterosexual orientations – so there's no excuse to not get yours!

For those of you with less time on your hands, there are a
number of quick activities throughout the book for a more
instant sexual fix. Be sure to tick off each activity after you do
it, and tally up your score at the back of the book to see where
your stock stands on the F-ing Frugal Exchange! The more
activities you do the more money you'll save and the more
sexy time you can clock on your hot and horny time sheet.

Whether you're funemployed, completely stagflated,
or a studied saver who's ready to flirt your way to the
frugal Olympics, it's time to cut up your credit cards,
slip into something a little more comfortable, and get
ready to Kama the Sutra out of this Recession.

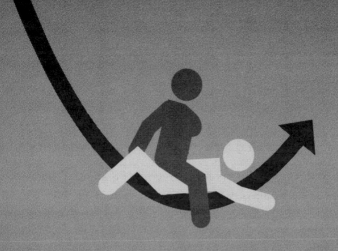

LONG-TERM INSEXMENTS

You've put your money where your bad-girl/boy mouth is and banked good and hard on a hottie. Make sure your investment pays off by tackling as many of these penny-saving activities as you can together. From home repairs and holiday plans, to date nights and driving to work, there's not a daily expense that can't be transformed into an affordable, tantalising treat for you and your partner. Not only will these activities keep your sex life on the up and down (and the in and out), you'll be richer and rosier by the day – trust me, your genitals are signing a cheque as you read this. So grab your partner and start investing, the sexy way.

HOME HARD-ONS AND PLEASURE GARDENS

Your home might be where your hard-on is, but that doesn't mean it's not costing you thousands every year. Turn DIY into DI 'oh my!' and fight off the recession (bondage straps optional) from behind closed doors.

Total Liquidity

**Get lathered like a hottie while savouring
every drop of your water bill.**

YOU WILL NEED:

- A hot and steamy shower
- Your favourite sexy-scented shower gel or soap

WHAT TO DO:

Yes, water costs money – we're not suggesting for a second
that you forego your daily cleanse, only that you make the
most of every drop of water, get cleaned up in the dirtiest
way possible and shower like a sex kitten. Turn the shower on
hot, let the room fill with steam, and then tell your partner to
come and help you fix something in the bathroom. Position
yourself provocatively under the hot water, while lathering
your body with your favourite shower gel or soap. When they
see you poised, and ready to unleash some serious shower-
certified sex moves, they won't be able to resist stripping off
and giving you the dirtiest scrub of your life. When you're

done, return the favour and make the most of the steam-filled room by going down on them until the air clears.

SEXONOMIC BONUS:

Lay some fluffy towels on the bathroom floor to soak up any wasted splashes and create some steam of your own by pulling your shower buddy down and riding them till you're hot, sweaty, and ready for another wash.

FRUGAL RATING:

You're getting wet (in all the right places) and sharing water. Saving the environment and your money in one hot and steamy session, good job!

Invisible Hands

Turn the lights down low and let your hands have all the fun for free!

YOU WILL NEED:

- A very dark room
- Candles (optional)

WHAT TO DO:

We love sex with the lights on, but there's no point paying extra on your electricity bill when the purse strings are already so tight. Turn all the lights in the house off, draw the blinds and let your imagination run wild when you can't even see your partner's face. Girls, put on your most provocative underwear, and boys show off your body in a cute pair of underpants and then play hide and seek in the dark for a truly electrifying sexual encounter. If you're seeking, locate your partner in the house and try to sneak up on them. As the seeker's reward your partner must strip for you, while touching their own body and describing everything they're doing to themselves and everything they want to do to you using the filthiest language they can muster. Try not to touch them during this time, but feel free to touch yourself. When you cannot control the urge any longer, then you can get in on the action by putting your hands all over their body in the pitch black. The darkness will add another level of mystery and imagination to your foreplay, and is ideal for character role-play and making the most of all your home's dirty little corners... and your own!

SEXONOMIC BONUS:

Scared of the dark? Light a few candles and position them around your house, leading your partner to whichever room you want to sex them up in. Every time they pass a candle they blow it out, and when they find you, you blow him or pleasure her as a reward.

FRUGAL RATING:

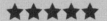

Turning the lights down low has never been so good for your wallet or your libido.

Privatised Porn Star

Role-play away the financial frustrations of getting things fixed with your own personal porn star.

YOU WILL NEED:

- A leaky pipe – preferably in the kitchen (just block the sink and leave the taps running for effect).
- Worker's overalls
- A tool kit (filled with sex toys and some heavy-duty lube)
- A skimpy negligee

WHAT TO DO:

Take a day off work, get dressed up in your most revealing bedroom attire, and phone your partner on their mobile phone. Tell them that the pipe is leaking in the kitchen and that you need them to come home from work to help you fix it. Leave some worker's overalls by the front door with a tool kit (put your favourite sex toys and stimulating lube in there so your partner cottons on to the game) and a note telling them to get dressed for work and meet you in the kitchen. From this moment forth, your partner is the hot plumber who asks, 'What seems to be the problem?' and you are the bored housewife/husband who can't wait to get their hands on the plumber's tools. Have your partner check out the sink, splash them with water so they're forced to strip off out of the overalls, and then proceed to flirt outrageously with them until they give in to the forbidden desire and seduce you. Make sure you tip them well for their service!

SEXONOMIC BONUS:

Play as hard to get as your time schedule allows and stay in character so your partner will want you even more. If you're not shy, and are feeling risky, leave the curtains open and get naked and naughty and risk giving the neighbours an eye-full!

FRUGAL RATING:

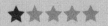

Let's be honest, you're still going to have to call a qualified plumber (or a cleaner after all that mess), but at least your own pipes got a thorough seeing to.

Reveal Your Assets

**Get your windows cleaned while turning
your lover's mind all kinds of dirty.**

YOU WILL NEED:

- Some mildly dirty windows with curtains
- A ladder
- A bucket
- A sponge

WHAT TO DO:

It's about time your partner stopped playing Xbox and did
some hard labour (don't worry, no one needs to have a baby
for this one, unless you plan it that way!) Promise them a good
bonking session if they clean the windows for you. Draw all the
curtains closed, hand them a bucket filled with soapy water,
a sponge, and get the ladder set up so all they have to do is
climb and scrub. Once they've started, head back inside and
position yourself in front of the window they're cleaning. Turn

on your favourite sexy tunes, pull back the curtains and dance seductively. Remove an item of clothing, and when their face is pressed up against the glass and they're starting to drool, pull the curtains shut and move to the next dirty window ready to reveal more. By the time your partner's finished soaping and squeegeeing, you should be naked and feeling horny from having their eyes all over you. When your personal window washer comes inside they'll be ready to come with you over and over again. Oh, and if you didn't distract them too much with your hotness, your windows should be clean! And if you're the brawny one in this relationship, then tell your partner you'll get up the ladder if they make it worth your while.

SEXONOMIC BONUS:

Getting your partner to do manual labour equals a high-five and a trip to your favourite clothes store (on sale day!) to find your next sexy strip-tease outfit. Windows don't stay clean forever, you know! And if you were the one doing the hard work, you deserve to spend those savings sipping a beer and getting your own private lap dance – from your partner!

FRUGAL RATING:

Super saving on home maintenance and hot and horny sex. It doesn't get better than that!

Dirty Sock Market

There'll be no more hunting for laundry change after trying this wet and wild wash cycle.

YOU WILL NEED:

- A basket of dirty laundry
- A freestanding washing machine (one you can sit on)

WHAT TO DO:

Yes, we know it's much easier to drop off your delicates at your local laundrette and leave the hard work to someone else, but service is costly, and that washing machine should start earning its keep. Drag your partner to wherever you keep your washer/dryer, make them watch you bend over and load up all your dirty laundry. Then, act surprised and tell them that you need to wash the clothes you're wearing. Strip off so you're standing there in nothing but your undies and finish loading up the washer. Turn it on and then make the most of how turned on they'll be by getting hot and heavy right there. Lift yourself or your partner up onto the washing machine while you go down on them or vice versa for extra vibrating goodness. If your laundry's done but you're not, throw it in the dryer and start all over again. You don't get that kind of service down at the laundrette.

SEXONOMIC BONUS:

If you keep this up, treat yourself to a drop-off laundry once a month, but keep your hottie's heart racing, and their face blushing, by throwing in a sexy thong or pair of briefs with their wash.

FRUGAL RATING:

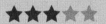

Make sure your clothes actually make it into the washer and that you don't break the machine with your hot and heavy laundry-day antics – it'll be hard explaining that one to your roommates/parents/the kind lady at the Laundrette.

Va-Va-Value Added

Say 'How you doin'?' to home repairs with this frisky way to DIY.

YOU WILL NEED:

- Some home repairs, preferably outdoors
- A sun lounger
- Sexy swimwear
- A tall, cool drink with ice cubes
- Overalls

WHAT TO DO:

Don't hire in help to finish the deck, use the brains and (hopefully some) brawn that lazes around your house all the time and get jobs done at no extra cost. Whether you need the fence painted, the lawn mowed or your favourite gazebo erected, ask your buffer half to get it done. Put on your sexiest swimwear and order them around the garden while seductively sliding ice cubes over your body. Tell them when they're finished sweating it out in the garden they can quench their thirst by licking your drink from your body. If you're the one who likes to do all the hard graft around your house, then simply make the bargain work in your favour.

SEXONOMIC BONUS:

Two pairs of wandering hands are better than one – get jobs done faster by stripping off and climbing into a pair of sweaty overalls too. Your hot-house help won't be able to keep their hands off you as you hammer, nail, and erect all kinds of hard and heavy things in your back garden.

FRUGAL RATING:

Home repairs are costly at the best of times, so make sure you get as much banging for your buck as possible.

Double Dip Impressions

Inject some colour into your home and some sexy time into your interiors.

YOU WILL NEED:

• A bucket of paint (go for something water-soluble that neither of you are allergic to – this is just for fun and no one likes an unsightly rash!)

• A cover for your floor

• A wall you want to decorate

• A ladder

WHAT TO DO:

No need to call in professional painter/decorators when you want to brighten up your home, instead save a fortune by suggesting a sexy DIY session with your partner. Use your hands to cover each other's bodies in the paint while kissing, then, when your partner's turned on and ready to decorate you, have them press the front of your body up hard against the bare wall, while touching, licking or penetrating you from behind. Roll around together and push their back up against the wall so you can go down on them, and then cover each other in more paint and repeat. For athletic decorators, use the ladder as a prop – ask your sex god or goddess to straddle it, pole dance with it, rest on it while they go down on you, and if you have the time, climb it to decorate up high. This wet, messy activity will leave your walls looking like amateur hour, but your inner walls or bulging brush feeling like they've had a thorough seeing to.

SEXONOMIC BONUS:

Reward your hard, hard work with a long, sexy soak in the bath – scrub each other good and proper to get rid of all that paint in hard to reach places.

FRUGAL RATING:

Your walls are going to look like a chimpanzee had his wicked way with a can of paint, so you might want to consider redecorating (with your clothes on) sometime soon.

Hello, Mr Bond

TV licenses are for boring people who aren't getting any. That's not you.

YOU WILL NEED:

- A sexy costume (think Bond girl/007, Lara Croft/ Jack Sparrow, Jessica Rabbit/Superman)
- Any props to bring your character to life

WHAT TO DO:

If you're watching TV with your partner, chances are you're not having sex. Pull the plug on your overpriced TV license and bid farewell to no-nookie nights by creating your own erotic programming schedule. Get your partner a drink and make sure they're sitting comfortably on the sofa. Give them a choice of sexy-sounding channels to choose from and then go get dressed up in an orgasm-inducing character costume from a TV show or movie. When you enter the living room, improvise a scene in character and involve your partner in the charade. Keep the role-play going as long as possible, before you finally can't help yourself and grab your partner on the sofa for some living room loving. There's no TV show on the planet that wraps its legs around you (or that will do things to your erogenous zones with its mouth), so we can guarantee your partner won't want to channel surf any time soon.

SEXONOMIC BONUS:

You might have cut yourselves off from the passion-killer that is TV, but that doesn't mean you can't enjoy a little audiovisual stimulation. Pick up a sexy flick or porn movie on DVD and enjoy even more intimacy for a fraction of the cost.

FRUGAL RATING:

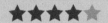

So long, farewell to costly TV bills, movie-night popcorn and Cokes and say hello to a far more intimate viewing experience.

Backwardation Relations

Scrub the dishes while your lover, um, scrubs your dishes.

Your dishwasher is rinsing away your cash flow, but doing the washing up is completely unsexy, right? Or so you thought! Tell your partner you'll do the dishes if they stand behind you and make it worth your while. With your hands elbow high in rubber gloves and greasy water, you'll be helpless to their advances. Wiggle your butt or flex your rock-hard cheeks to draw them close and then try to scour that baking tin clean while your partner teases your nipples, thrusts their hand inside your underwear and finally pulls off your clothes and does sexy things to you from behind. We bet that from now on you'll be making a full-on roast every Sunday, so the washing up takes all afternoon.

KEEPING IT UP
APPEARANCES

It's no surprise that you and your partner spend your disposable incomes on new clothes, beauty products, and stylish gadgets – just look at you, you're gorgeous, but do you remember the last time someone went down on you at the mall or you orgasmed while trying on a new (overpriced) dress or designer suit? Exactly. Try out these activities and enjoy fashion and beauty while getting yours.

Trim the Hedge Fund

You may be poor, but an overgrown bush is more a sign of laziness than poverty.

YOU WILL NEED:

- A well-grown hedge (of the lady/man-garden variety)
- Your preferred hair removal equipment
- Accessories of your choice – glitter, vajazzle jewels, leaves, etc.

WHAT TO DO:

Although it's quite the delight to have a complete stranger tear the roots (and your very soul) from your hairy love zone (or your partner's), you will always pay a premium for professional service and at times like these cutting back is the only way you can afford to get a down-there haircut. Trim that hedge on the cheap and reap the rewards of frugality, by insisting your partner has to give you the trim and treatment you desire – if you like your bush bushy then insist on doing theirs instead. Make it clear that if they want to see your noo-noo looking its best (or if they want theirs to dazzle), they have to do the dirty work themselves or let you show of your topiary skills. Make sure whoever's going to be removing the hair is fully briefed and that they have all the DIY tools of the trade they require. Guaranteed whether you're tidying up their garden or they're mowing yours, you'll both have so much fun the recipient will soon be asking for a quick tidy up on a regular basis. Although it may not be the life you're both accustomed to, the private gardener is sure to get turned on after giving their lover's hedge the royal treatment.

SEXONOMIC BONUS:

Make sure whoever's doing all the hard labour takes a break and has their tackle treated to some attention of its own, as a reward for stripping the other person bare and saving cash.

FRUGAL RATING:

This might not be the pain-free experience you/ they hoped for, and you're still going to have to fork out for all the essentials, but it beats being broke or walking around with a brimming bush.

Boom and Bust

AKA how to get your lover in the mood without spending a fortune on sexy undies.

YOU WILL NEED:

- A shopping centre
- A willing partner
- An ounce of confidence

WHAT TO DO:

Sexy silky bras, lace-trimmed panties and tight Calvin Kleins are the aphrodisiac of the wealthy. Why waste your time picking out sultry suspenders, come-to-bed corsets or burly boxers if you partner's just going to rip them off to get to the good stuff? Follow these simple instructions and achieve the same titillating effect without spending a thing. Take your partner to the nearest shopping centre and head straight to an underwear shop or lingerie department. Walk around the shop together picking out all the sexiest and most expensive items you can find (for him, for her, or for yourself), telling them how hot they are and how naughty they or you will look in them. Head to the changing room to try them on (or get cozy in the waiting area if your partner is more in the purchasing mood) and have your partner sit on one of those little chairs just outside. Whichever one of you is trying on clothes gets dressed up in each ensemble, and then stands in the entrance to the changing room so their partner can see how hot they look. (If this is out of either of your comfort zones, then just flash a shoulder, leg or booty shot from the dressing room door.) Politely hand all the items back after you're done and head to the next shop. Before your parking ticket is up you'll both be ready to hop in the car and drive home for some post-window-shopping sex.

SEXONOMIC BONUS:

If your partner can't stand to watch from afar, sneak them into the dressing room for some personal assistance (or head in yourself if your partner is the one dressing up all sexy). Just don't blame us if you get banned from buying undies there forever!

FRUGAL RATING:

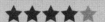

Parking ticket aside (and maybe a quick drink in the food court) this freebie gets you all the results without any of the shopper's remorse.

Blow Out

Wash and blow-dries blowing your budget? Why not suck, blow and lick your partner instead?

YOU WILL NEED:

- A full head of hair (baldies need not apply)
- Your favourite shampoos and conditioners
- A bath
- A shower/water jug
- Scented candles

WHAT TO DO:

There's nothing sexy about heading to the hairdresser – a bunch of loud-mouthed stylists or miserable barbers nattering about how good the weather was in Ibiza or the latest footie scores is a complete kick in the libido. Stop spending your wages on overpriced rinses and extortionate blow-dries and get that hair washed while a naked hottie massages you from behind. Dress up the bathroom in candlelit wonderment and fill the bath with hot soapy water. Climb in and then invite your own personal stylist into the bathroom and let them squeeze in behind you, their legs enveloping your hips. Ask them to rinse your hair (either using a shower attachment or a simple water jug), touching them while they get to work, and then massage in the shampoo, rinse and repeat with conditioner (of course). Keep them entertained with your hands and your body, but make sure you get your money's worth before you start splashing around like a pair of horny dolphins.

SEXONOMIC BONUS:

All great hairdressers deserve a tip for their time. Rather than wait for a blow dry from your stylist, put a towel on the bathroom floor, get down on your knees and give them the best oral sex ever as a thank you.

FRUGAL RATING:

Your partner might not be a natural with a pair of straightening irons but you're never going to get that kind of service, no matter where you get your hair done.

Hot Trading

Think Julia Roberts in *Pretty Woman* (after she's transformed from being a hooker into being a Beverly Hills beauty).

YOU WILL NEED:

- A group of awesome and willing friends
- A living room
- A bunch of old but sexy clothes you don't want any more
- A couple of bottles of wine

WHAT TO DO:

Throwing a Sexy Swap is all about replacing those 'wear it once' negligees and 'when I was ten pounds lighter' slinky dresses and getting new ones without paying a penny. Invite all your girl (or well-dressed guy) friends to the swap at your house. Tell people to bring a bag full of unwanted clothes (or more!). The only criteria are that they be gorgeous, sexy, sassy, and clean. When they arrive at the swap they throw all their unwanted clothes into the middle of the room and are invited to try on anything from the growing pile and take home what they want. Crack open a couple of bottles of wine to help ease self-conscious people and before you know it everyone will be swapping sex stories and taking home a whole bag full of gorgeous new clothes. Make sure you throw everything into a hot wash (who knows what your friends have been up to!) and then take your favourite ensemble out with your partner on date night. If you're a guy and aren't into skimpy negligees, you could help your partner set up a clothes swap (you're sure to enjoy the results) and be the sexy server at the swapping soiree.

SEXONOMIC BONUS:

Spend some of the money you saved not buying that costly outfit for Valentine's Day by treating your partner to a takeaway or a nice bottle of wine.

FRUGAL RATING:

Not only have you eliminated the need for a sexy clothes shopping budget for quite a while, you've got your partner turned on and reused a whole pile of unwanted clothes. You're like a sexy, green financial guru!

Full-On FTSE

While the FTSE's down why not get comfortable and ask your lover to really rub it in?

YOU WILL NEED:

- A strong pair of hands
- Two tired and weary feet
- Massage oil, if it pleases you

WHAT TO DO:

Your feet are all kinds of erogenous and if you thought they weren't they will be after this recession-ready activity. Yes, there is something truly decadent about the uncalloused hands of a professional masseuse/masseur. But if you or your partner are good with your digits in the bedroom, combine that with a little rhythm and pressure (two things you're both already well practised in) because it's time to throw caution to the wind, throw off your shoes and take turns propping your little piggies up on each other's laps for some R&R. Enjoy watching each other moan with pleasure as you both try your hardest to make each other's feet feel divine. And why stop there? Surreptitiously remove items of your clothing when it's your turn to get toe-rubbed saying, 'Oh, it's a bit warm in here, isn't it?' until you're practically naked in front of your masseuse/masseur. Choose a body part, chuck them the massage oil, and Bob's your extremely horny uncle. Voila – your own personal full-body massage from the comfort of your couch.

SEXONOMIC BONUS:

If rubbing scented oil into your soft, supple skin (and your partner's) doesn't put a smile on both your faces, ask your partner to plant their face in the couch, straddle their back and give them a mounted massage they won't forget in a hurry.

FRUGAL RATING:

No awkward silences with Enya playing in the background and lots of slippery skin to skin contact with the right kind of friction. Minimum spend, maximum pleasure!

QUICK WIN TO GET IT IN

Treasury Chest

Enjoy sparkling from head to pelvis no matter how much you're in the red.

Let's face it, you're not going to be shopping at Tiffany's any time soon (for yourself, or for your partner), but diamonds – real or not – will always be a girl's best friend and a boy's most rewarded financial investment, whatever the economic climate. Pick up some edible and dazzling cake decorating treats (gold leaf, silver baubles, edible sparkly confetti) and something delicious and sticky – honey, chocolate spread, or tube icing works perfectly – and make the most of a boring mid-week evening by covering your bodies in glittery gems, affixed with your sticky substance of choice, and then licking and nibbling them off of each other's skin. You'll feel so decadent, delicious, and dirty covered in these titillating treasures that a trip to Tiffany's will be the last thing on your mind.

GET YOUR SEXY SWEAT ON

You still want to pay fifty quid a month to hang out in a stinky gym when you can give your abs, arms, and glutes a super sexy workout by jumping and humping one another when you walk in the door? We didn't think so. Oh, and this way your love muscles get a workout too. Total body conditioning at a fraction of the cost.

Stretch the Budget

It's called hot yoga, so there must be something hot about it, right?

YOU WILL NEED:

- A yoga studio, preferably Bikram
- A yoga mat, because that's not the kind of sweat you want to share with strangers
- A sexy yoga outfit

WHAT TO DO:

Yoga isn't just for yummy mummies and hippy folk who smell like swamps. Ordinary people should be able to afford to go to low-lit, scented rooms and stretch like celebrities, too. But it's impossible to justify the extortionate cost of lying on a mat and being told off for your incorrect attempt at Happy Baby pose when the price of bread keeps going up and up. Fortunately, most studios do first-time-is-free classes. Take advantage and make a date together for some hot yoga

(Bikram is best). Dress in your most flattering and fabulous workout clothes and position yourselves next to or in front of each other during the class. You are going to sweat like crazy, whilst looking completely serene, so make sure you give each other an eyeful every time you do Downward Facing Dog and you'll have doggy style on your lover's mind until you get back home and strip off for a shower.

SEXONOMIC BONUS:

Sweaty, invigorated and ready to romp after yoga?
Before you go home to bonk, treat yourselves
to a refreshing smoothie filled with healthy fruit
and veggies so you can go at it for hours!

FRUGAL RATING:

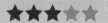

Unless you live in a large metropolis you're going to
run out of yoga studios willing to shell out free passes
pretty quickly. Worst case scenario, pump up the
heat at home and get posing in your living room.

Ponzi Steam

Always thought of public pools as cesspits for germs and annoying old people and a good place to contract a foot fungus? Think again.

YOU WILL NEED:

- Your sexiest swimwear
- A local leisure centre with steam or sauna facilities

WHAT TO DO:

Your local leisure centre is probably the furthest from your mind as a romantic location – crowds of annoying teenagers, miserable oldies who cause gridlock in the 'fast' lanes. Point taken, but lots of public pools have saunas and steam rooms ideal for getting hot, horny and indulging in some forbidden heavy petting at a fraction of the cost of membership-only gyms. Call in advance and find out which time of day is quietest (the last hour before closing in the evening is often a good choice) and head to the pool. Make the most of your money and get your blood pumping by doing a few laps with your partner – groping each other every time you stop for a breather. Head to the steam room or sauna when they're empty and sit close. When the coast is clear think hand job and give your partner a good feel-up whilst nobody's looking. Keep your eyes on the door – the risk of being caught will only add to the excitement!

SEXONOMIC BONUS:

You've probably worked up an appetite in your stomach and your by now lubed-up love parts, so pick up some nosh on the way home and feed each other while your relaxed, chlorine-scented bodies cuddle close on the sofa and prepare for the second lap.

FRUGAL RATING:

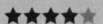

A few quid for a work out and an orgasm?
Now that's value for money!

Stick or Twister

Who knew *Twister* could get so hot and sticky?

YOU WILL NEED:

- The game *Twister*
- A layered outfit that incorporates as many pieces as possible

WHAT TO DO:

Strictly speaking, *Twister* isn't a sport, but it is a physical activity, which, if played according to these guidelines will leave you sweaty and panting like a sexually relieved Olympian. Get your *Twister* set ready and layer on your clothes – you want to wear just enough that the anticipation of getting you naked will drive your partner wild. Play the game as usual, stretching and squirming to make sure your hands and feet stay on all the right spots. If your partner spots your hands or feet move from their designated spots then they get to select an item of your clothing that you have to remove. Play until one of you is completely naked – the player who has the most clothes left on is the winner. Pushing your flexibility to the max will leave your bendy body in perfect shape for a romp, and you're naked anyway, so why not?

SEXONOMIC BONUS:

As a reward for their lithe performance, whoever wins the game of *Twister* gets to choose the position you must be in for the victory romp!

FRUGAL RATING:

Providing you already own *Twister* this is good, wholesome, family fun on the cheap – minus the kids and double the kinks.

Vertical Equity

The great outdoors is just waiting to be explored and exploited. Put on your hiking boots and go and get frisky in the wild.

YOU WILL NEED:

- A pair of comfortable walking shoes/boots
- A suitable walking outfit
- A flask of hot tea
- A blanket

WHAT TO DO:

There's nothing like doing it outdoors to make you feel alive. Stop whinging on the Stairmaster, pack a Thermos, a blanket, and don your sexiest walking attire for a day in the countryside. Find a manageable hill with a well-marked walking trail and set off together. Hold hands as you walk and really enjoy each other's fully-clothed company. Talking about your favourite sexual experiences together will get you in the mood for what comes next. Once you've made it to the top of the mountain (OK, hill...) you've certainly earned yourself a quick wilderness romp. Make sure no one's around, find a thicket, and 'make hay while the sun shines'. If you're feeling frisky, and it's not too cold, lay down the blanket and go at it like wild animals. After you're done, be sure to remove any errant twigs from each other's hair and head back to the car for a much-needed rest and a cup of tea from your flask.

SEXONOMIC BONUS:

All that outdoor time and calorie-crunching activity will definitely have earned you a big meal and a pint. Head to a local country pub for a much-needed fill-me-up. No, not that kind, you dirty walkers!

FRUGAL RATING:

If there's a nip-ple in the air, give them a well-earned squeeze. Free country walks, thick bushes, and outdoor sex enthusiasts make a wonderful combination.

Under Water

Don't be shy – make a splash in your birthday suits for a wetter time!

YOU WILL NEED:

- Swimming attire (if you're not the nudist type)
- A secluded beach or lake
- A towel to dry each other off

WHAT TO DO:

Doing it in a pool will probably only draw looks of disgust and unfriendly references to *Showgirls* but making the most of the lubricated loveliness of natural bodies of water is a completely different matter. Drive out to a secluded spot (or make the most of this activity when you're camping), either by the beach or a lake. Skinny dipping is the sexiest way to go, so strip off and launch yourself into the water with your partner. Unless you're planning on a sneaky budget busting trip to the Caribbean any time soon, chances are the water will be cold. Cuddle together and rub each other's bodies to get the blood flowing. Find a spot where you're out of sight (unless you like it when people watch!) and make like octopi. Grab each other's freezing cold buttocks and pull yourselves close together. If you've got the stamina, have sex and don't stop until you're starting to sweat in the icy water. Burn those calories, baby, burn!

SEXONOMIC BONUS:

Warm off by a camp fire or BBQ, wrapped up in your towels or a blanket. As a cheap reward feed each other toasted marshmallows until you get a sugar rush and want to do it all over again.

FRUGAL RATING:

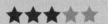

If you're pretty much landlocked, apart from a muddy looking city river, you might have to make quite a journey to find that lush lake or beautiful beach. If you have a hot tub in your back garden, then that might be a cheaper and warmer way to get this kind of underwater love.

QUICK WIN TO GET IT IN

2 for the Price of 1

Celebrity workouts might get you sweaty, but they're never going to turn you on too.

Tell your partner that you want to try out a new workout DVD. Entice them by saying it's hosted by all the girls/boys from *Hollyoaks*, or by an intense cage fighter (whatever will get them interested). Instead, pick up a porn movie that gets you hot and pop it in the DVD player. When the movie comes on tell your partner they'd better copy what's happening on the screen. Keep your eyes on the TV and do everything one of the actors is doing: strip when they strip, squeal when they squeal, and hopefully come when they come. Soon you'll be working up a sweat to rival any fitness instructor while yelping in ecstasy like an excited puppy.

CHEAP AND DIRTY DATE NIGHTS

Sick of pricey dinners and disappointing movies? A romantic getaway, expensive gift, or extravagant day of activities can leave you broke without always getting the bonk you'd hoped for at the end of the date. So don't pay through the nose to show your partner a good time – try out these cost-cautious activities that all lead to lots of heavy petting and date-night dirty and flirty behaviour.

Federal Reservations

When fine dining is out of your budget, dress up and indulge each other at home.

YOU WILL NEED:

- Supplies for a three-course dinner
- A black bow-tie and white undies for him
- A sexy black dress for her
- Some classical music
- Candles

WHAT TO DO:

There's nothing hotter than feeding each other fancy French delights you can't pronounce in a candlelit dining room full of quiet conversation, followed by dancing and dessert. But in real life, these places don't exist, and if they do they are usually full of old people and smell of cabbage. Reserve a table at Chez Vous and dine together *à deux*. Set the mood with candles and classical music. Get dressed up in your fine serving attire – girls, you get to wear a slinky black number, and guys, you can show off your muscles in a pair of tight white underpants and a black bow-tie – and take it in turns to serve each other the courses (joining each other to eat them, of course). Enjoy your dinner, and then stand up and hold each other close for a romantic dance, pressed together, skin-on-skin. Stay classy as long as you can take it and then slip out of your regalia and suggest that you take your dessert to the bedroom to eat it off each other's naked bodies (a chocolate mousse is ideal and delicious).

Bon appétit!

SEXONOMIC BONUS:

It's quite the feat to recreate the mood of a fancy restaurant in your kitchen, so as a reward for your efforts, get back into your clothes – guys, you might want more than just the bow-tie – and head out to a cocktail bar for a round of luxurious drinks if you're not too tired from any 'inter-course' activity.

FRUGAL RATING:

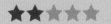

Making a nice meal doesn't come cheap (and it's not like you're going to serve each other beans on toast) but three courses at your place is definitely going to save you money over going out, and at least you can tip your waiter or waitress in a currency older than cash.

Titillating Tea Party

**All the fun of a scandalous tea party without any
of the financial complications.**

YOU WILL NEED:

- A secluded park
- A picnic blanket
- Finger food
- Iced tea (with an alcoholic edge, if you prefer)
- Water pistols

WHAT TO DO:

Tea parties are not just for conservative politicians and six-
year-old girls. Spike some iced tea (or pick up some Pimm's),
pack a hamper if you have one, and head to your nearest park
for a loved-up, boozy afternoon. Find a spot that's shady and
secluded and laze on your picnic blanket, lying in each other's
arms. Enjoy each other's company and each other's bodies;
run your fingers slowly up and down each other's arms and

bare stomachs. Feed each other strawberries, sandwiches, salads and sweets from the hamper and slowly sip away at the alcohol until you're light-headed and feeling horny. Don't ruin the day by getting arrested, but fondle and frolic with each other enough that there's tent-pitching or damp patches of the erotic variety and you're both wishing home was a lot closer. To cool off, pull out the water guns and chase each other around the park. But, beware, the sight of each other's nipples, standing to attention under your soaked T-shirts, might be more than you can stand. Pack up your picnic and head home (or to the car) for adult-only entertainment.

SEXONOMIC BONUS:

If it's hot and you're horny, a great way to cool off without losing that lovin' feeling is with an ice lolly. Buy one from the ice-cream van, and then suck on it till your partner's wishing they were a frozen fruity snack.

FRUGAL RATING:

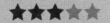

You get frugal high-fives for packing your own picnic and entertaining each other with your hands (free), some snacks (almost free) and a good old-fashioned water fight (free and extremely fun!)

Bank Roll in the Hay

There's nothing like seeing other animals humping to make you want to do it yourself.

YOU WILL NEED:

- A local farm that welcomes volunteers (city farm, children's farm, etc.)
- A pair of welly boots

WHAT TO DO:

You're not the only one who would like to be taken roughly in a barn. Fulfill that dream by finding a farm near to you that allows volunteers to come and help feed the animals and tend to crops – there are lots of great city farms, animal sanctuaries and children's petting zoos that welcome volunteers (although they might not be expecting the bend-me-over-and-do-me help that you're offering). Get all dressed down in your wellies and take each other on a day trip to the farm. As you sweat and toil over cute goats or giant cucumbers, keep your eyes peeled for unattended sheds, barns and haystacks. When the supervisors are out of sight, sneak to this secluded spot, give each other a hand (in the right places). Bend over (preferably against a bale of hay) and go for a bit of rough and ready right there. The dirt and sweat from the day will only make it hotter, and the quickie nature will have you coming in your wellies. Nice work, Farmer Giles.

SEXONOMIC BONUS:

After a hard day's farming and fondling, head to a country pub nearby for a hearty dinner fit for all the work you and your partner put in.

FRUGAL RATING:

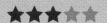

Treating yourself to a pub lunch loses you a few points here, but you're going to need it after cuddling all those cute animals and the effort it will take to get the straw out of your bales.

Sin-terest Free Loan

Turn that sexy-geek fantasy into a libido-loving reality.

YOU WILL NEED:

- A valid library card
- A pair of sexy but studious glasses
- A fitted A-line skirt or suit
- A white shirt (buttoned a little too low)
- Killer heels for girls

WHAT TO DO:

If you're the kind of lover who associates libraries with hours spent fantasising over the hottie from your sociology lectures then this is the game for you. Cast caution to the wind, seize your library card from a dusty crevice of your wallet, and get tarted up in your favourite sexy-geek outfit (skirts and shirts for girls, and scruffy suits for boys). Don't forget the geek-chic glasses that scream 'I'm smart, but I like it dirty.' Text your partner to meet you at the library (NB: check they know where the library is if it's been a while). When they arrive, stay out of sight, and pretend to peruse the shelves – they'll be looking for regular you, not über-hot geeky you, so this should be easy. If it's a big library, they might text you asking where the hell you are. Respond with lines like 'I'm being a naughty nerd in the kids' section.' or 'Getting all hot and bothered in cookery.' When they find you, drag them to the cosiest, quietest corner of the library, and without saying a word, put your hands down their pants or up their skirt and give them a warm welcome that will have your bookshelf-shy lover returning to the library week after week.

SEXONOMIC BONUS:

Before you leave, make the most of the library's facilities by heading to the sexual health section and selecting a few sex tips/position books. Peruse them together, while you start mentally undressing each other, then take them home and get down to business.

FRUGAL RATING:

The library is a great place to get kinky while picking up a bit of free sex advice. Soft lighting, quiet corners, and the thrill of doing something a little naughty somewhere so conservative, will set your pulses racing. Try to keep the noise down – house rules!

Piggy Bonk

Put your pennies in a pig and save up for a date night extravaganza full of pent-up excitement.

YOU WILL NEED:

- A piggy bank
- Spare change
- A lot of self-control

WHAT TO DO:

Splashing out on a fancy night out can be costly: new outfit, haircut or shave, dinner, drinks, cab to snog in on the way home... Times might be tough, but that doesn't mean you shouldn't have some fancy fun. Use a piggy bank to save up together for a weekly, monthly or annual date (obviously the longer you save for the more phenomenal the date could be!). To make saving a little more enjoyable, set a list of tariffs with mini rewards you or your partner get if they donate their cash to the tin. And with treats like this, you'll have saved up for a kinky weekend in Paris in no time!

If they donate...

£1 = they get a take-me-to-bed-and-do-dirty-things-to-me kiss

£5 = you must perform a striptease for them

£10 = your mouth goes anywhere they want for at least 10 minutes

£20 = you tie them up and do unspeakable things to them

Remember, this is a game for both of you to play! So get saving and enjoy some of life's free and frisky pleasures.

SEXONOMIC BONUS:

Saving doesn't have to take forever. Put the pressure on and see how much you can entice each other to donate in one week and then use some of the money to do one of this book's more costly activities.

FRUGAL RATING:

Spend no money, save even more. You might enjoy this activity so much that you'll end up paying off your next holiday off the back of your naughty behaviour.

QUICK WIN TO GET IT IN

Exchange Dates

Double the dating; double the turn-on; half the price.

There's nothing like seeing your partner flirting outrageously with someone else to drive you wild with desire. Invite a couple of friends (or another couple, as long as there is a hottie for each of you to flirt with) out for drinks. Remember, because there are four of you everything will be cheaper. Share appetisers, bottles of wine and cab rides to make the night super affordable. Spend the whole night flirting with everyone but your partner, especially the other guy/girl in your group, and make sure your partner does the same – be sure to catch your partner's eye every so often to check you're both having a good time. As the night draws to a close you'll be missing each other's eyes on your bodies and their lips on your neck that you'll be hungry for each other and ready to pounce as soon as you get home. Don't know any hot, flirt-worthy couples? Never fear. This works equally well if you head to a bar, pub or club and each of you choose a stranger to flirt outrageously with.

FUN FEEDS AND PRIMAL NEEDS

Food, glorious food. The relationship between eating with our mouths and feasting with our genitals is so close that it would be foolish to think you couldn't combine the oral pleasures of both to create some belly-stuffing, libido-loving activities that give your bank balance room to breathe.

Shovel Ready

Get into the self-sufficient spirit and you'll soon understand why the baby boomer generation occurred.

YOU WILL NEED:

- A garden (failing that, some window boxes)
- Vegetable seeds
- Gardening tools (trowel, watering can, gloves, etc.)

WHAT TO DO:

When you can't afford to eat, a garden can be your best friend as well as a source of some serious sexual urges. Dig up that useless patch of grass and fill it with the Earth's bounty as a couple. Make gardening a weekly event, and schedule it right before a refreshing shower together to wash off all the sweat and dirt. There are no rules about how dirty you can get in the garden, but below are a few Recession Kama Sutra ideas for spicing up your shovel time.

- Girls, at regular intervals, bend over to plant some seeds and all he'll be thinking about is planting his seed in you

- Guys, stiffen up that love muscle to use as a dibber for planting bulbs

- Girls, go braless in the garden, Charlie Dimmock style, and your partner won't be able to keep their eyes off you

- Guys, make sure you do all the heavy lifting (shirtless) so your partner can admire your rippling muscles and sweaty body while you work

- Girls, stake the shovel in the ground and pole dance around it

- Both: get muddy and have a tickle fight

SEXONOMIC BONUS:

When your first veggies emerge from the earth, create a meal with them accompanied by a lovely bottle of wine to toast your self-sufficient success.

FRUGAL RATING:

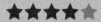

Gardens (like the lady variety) are the creation that keeps on giving. And like achieving orgasm, sometimes it can involve a lot of effort, but the ultimate result is always worth it.

Big Mac Index

Intense salt, sugar and a dirty drive-through gets your pulse racing at a reasonable price.

YOU WILL NEED:

- A burger chain drive-through
- A car
- An unhealthy appetite

WHAT TO DO:

If fast food were sex it would be a hot and dirty quickie behind a bike shed. Indulge your inner burger junkie, pile in the car with your partner, and head to the nearest drive-through. Super-size this cheap thrill by keeping each other's intimate bits entertained the minute you get in line. Whether his hand is doing the work between her chicken nuggets or her lips are locked around his hotdog, you'll struggle with anticipation as you place your order and make your way to the pick-up window. Be sure to regain composure before your order is up; otherwise the ketchup isn't going to be the only red thing in the car. Drive to a secluded spot or motorway lay-by and give in to whichever instinct is more overwhelming – the desire to chow down on greasy fries and cheesy burgers or the desire to crawl on top of each other and ride each other into the sunset. Choose the latter and you'll have a lovely lukewarm feast to finish up with.

SEXONOMIC BONUS:

If you manage to make one another come before the nice lady hands you your burgers, drive back round again and treat yourselves to a milkshake, because that, my dears, is thirsty work.

FRUGAL RATING:

Those burgers may come cheap, but with the sugar, salt and sexy times included, you're going to be so hooked on this drive-through the voice through the speaker will start saying, 'Your usual?'

Credit Crunch Cramdown

Welcome to the all-you-can-eat buffet that guarantees a good time.

YOU WILL NEED:

- A selection of your favourite foods, homemade and ready to eat
- Two plates
- Two forks

WHAT TO DO:

The all-you-can-eat experience is a little like sex. Yes, you can completely stuff yourself until you are unable to move, but it's equally pleasurable to resist temptation and just have a little taste of everything. Make enough food to last a few meals and then fill each other's plates with a generous helping of all the goodies you've prepared. Sit close and feed the food to each other, slowly and sensually, so you both savour each mouthful and really taste your food. You'll be so involved with each other, in a short time the piles of food will become secondary to the lips and eyes of the person feeding it to you. Bite into ripe strawberries together, let your tongue linger over a sip of wine, suck on a spoonful of chocolate mousse, and before long you'll be nibbling on an ear, licking a warm neck and sucking on appendages. Toss your napkins aside, grab your glasses of wine and finish this meal off in the bedroom. When you come back to the table a few hours later, you'll have enough food to keep this game going for a few more nights.

SEXONOMIC BONUS:

Your restraint is admirable and should be rewarded. If you have the post-coital munchies, share a generous helping of dessert on the sofa, in the bedroom or lying right there on the dining room floor where you gave in to a much cheaper form of temptation.

FRUGAL RATING:

Food's not going to come cheap, and neither should you. By showing restraint both at the table and in the sack you will have a much deeper, more pleasurable and longer-lasting enjoyment of your dinner and your date.

Stimulus Lunch Package

It's like at school when your mum packed you a lunch, only dirtier, and nothing to do with your mum.

YOU WILL NEED:

- Two lunchboxes (it doesn't have to be of the Disney variety – a simple Tupperware will do)
- Post-it notes
- Lunch supplies

WHAT TO DO:

Heading out for a gourmet sandwich or a long pub lunch with colleagues can be fun, but buying out five times a week is an unnecessary cost that's not doing your bank balance (or your sex drive) any favours. Stock up at home with delicious and healthy snacks and prepare a lunch for each other every night before bed (or before work in the morning). Fill your

Tupperware boxes with tasty treats, but before packing them in your bags, you must both write a fun and flirty message for your partner on a Post-it note and stick it to their lunchbox. When they get the midday munchies and fish their pack out for a nibble, the first thing they'll see is a sweet and sexy or downright dirty one-liner from you to enjoy with their meal. Instead of heading out to the greasy spoon or local drive-through, which will leave your bellies bloated and sex drive heading south, the healthy and wholesome snacks will give you the energy you'll need for the sex marathon that's waiting for you both when you get back home.

SEXONOMIC BONUS:

Once a week treat each other to something extra special in your lunchboxes – a bar of luxurious dark chocolate or a bag of their favorite high-end snack – as a reward for saving so much money and turning each other on.

FRUGAL RATING:

You are going to save a fortune, probably drop a few pounds and think about sex even more than before. Win, win, win!

QUICK WIN TO GET IT IN

Salivating and Satisficing

Detract attention from unsavoury cheap dinners by making them in the buff.

If you're living off ramen noodles and tins of no-brand baked beans then you know that times are tough (or you're living with a student). But just because your stomach is suffering, it doesn't mean your love life has to. You may not be able to afford libido-loving oysters, but if you strip off and stir those beans wearing nothing but an apron, then your grateful partner won't be able to keep their hands off you. Take it in turns to make dinner in the buff and you'll soon be glad you're not in the midst of an extravagant culinary creation when that apron gets whipped off and you are ravished right there on the kitchen floor. And the best thing about beans is, they taste just as good reheated, after your heart rate has returned to normal.

TAKE A BREAK
AND BONK WHILE
BEING BROKE

If you're the type that needs that getaway to get it on, fear not. Just because your money is taking a break of its own it doesn't mean you don't deserve a time-out and some hot and horny holiday sex. Whether you vacate, staycate or just stay at home, there's a holiday to be had and a hottie to hump.

Sexy Staycation

You don't have to go far away to get away from it all and reignite the flames of passion.

YOU WILL NEED:

- A tent and car or caravan
- A campsite
- Camping gear – stove, sleeping bags, etc.
- Marshmallows
- A bottle of something strong (optional)

WHAT TO DO:

Yes, that trip to an exotic island would have been amazing, but even with 1-star hotels and budget air fares a trip abroad is still a pretty poor investment with the economy looking so rocky. Make the decision to stay at home and take your pick from hundreds of beautiful countryside campsites for a romantic staycation. Whether you're a glamping novice or an outdoorsy pro, spending a few nights out in the open air, nestled together under the stars, fondling each other through your sleeping bags, is a great way to reconnect mentally and more importantly, physically, with your lover. Light a camp fire and toast marshmallows to feed to each other, take long, quiet walks along bridleways and rivers (dipping into the hedgerow for some frisky foraging), and get an early night when the sun goes down with a bottle of something strong. Once you're inside your canvas cocoon, you will be freeing yourselves from your sleeping bags so you can hump the sunset away, scare off the foxes with your own pleasurable howls, and stay warm together well into the night.

SEXONOMIC BONUS:

By saving your sexy selves a fortune on transportation and accommodation, you'll have a little spare cash to blow at the local watering hole. Locate it on your last night, do shots and stumble back to the tent like seasoned campers.

FRUGAL RATING:

Holidays are optional, but with so little to do and so much time to kill in the great outdoors (especially if it rains) you'll end up spending most of your time rolling around on your ground sheet without spending a thing.

Loved Up Lock-In

Turn your home into a hotel for a relaxing weekend that actually saves you money.

YOU WILL NEED:

- Food for two days
- Movies (erotic, if you prefer)
- Reading materials (sex tips, magazines, etc.)
- Massage oil
- Alcohol (or other beverages if you don't drink)

WHAT TO DO:

Nothing. No, really. The aim of this activity is to turn what is seemingly an ordinary weekend into a romantic getaway where you don't go anywhere. Turn off your mobile phones, computers, internet, etc. and transform your house into a hotel. You arrive on Saturday morning, waking up together in your comfortable bed. Lounge around all day, eating delicious food, drinking wine, massaging each other, dancing to your favourite music... the list is endless. The one rule of the activity is you're never allowed to leave the house (the garden, if you have one, is not off limits). Spend the entire weekend disconnected from your lives and reconnected to each other, the way you would if you were strolling through Paris, cycling the canals of Amsterdam or relaxing on a boat on the French Riviera. Keep things interesting with erotic movies in the evening, and by trying out bendy sex moves you've never attempted.

SEXONOMIC BONUS:

If you manage to spend the whole weekend enjoying the home you already have and all the places you can shag each other senseless, then take Monday off work, and head to one of your favourite local spots for a picnic/pub lunch/activity and some well-earned outdoors time.

FRUGAL RATING:

What sounds like a lazy weekend in is actually a cheap challenge that forces you to spend time exploring each other, rather than an exotic location. Great for your wallets and even better for your body.

Euro Love Zone

**Can't afford to take a trip to the continent?
Recreate the romance in your own back garden.**

You will need access to:

- A French restaurant
- A lake with boating rentals
- A free art gallery
- A bowling alley

And girls (or fun and flexible guys) will need:

- A corset
- Fishnet tights
- A large frilly skirt

WHAT TO DO:

Paris has long been the destination for lovers, proposals and
honeymoons, but that kind of continental luxury doesn't come
cheap. Plan a week of whimsical France-inspired dates with your

partner that will get you in the mood for love, ooh la la-style! On Monday, set the mood at a local French restaurant. The meal, the wine, and hopefully the cheesy French music will get you all ready and roused for the rest of the week. Tuesday (weather depending) take a boat out on a lake/river in your area. Flirt your way around a free art gallery on Wednesday, and then head to a bowling club or alley (or boules tournament if you can find one) on Thursday for some ball-tossing antics. Finish off the week on Friday with a private Moulin Rouge show in your bedroom. Girls, do the can-can for your partner wearing fishnets, a corset, and a ruffled skirt, and boys, your Eiffel Tower will be standing tall and ready to climb in no time. Guy-guy couples can still get in on the Parisian pageantry even if they don't fancy wearing the frilly skirt!

SEXONOMIC BONUS:

You can-can have a fanciful, flirty French time without all the unnecessary expense, and as a reward you should definitely pick up some fancy French dessert and wine to enjoy over the weekend.

FRUGAL RATING:

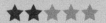

It's not cheap going out five nights in a row, but all the romance-inspired sex you'll be getting will be worth the effort. If you want to save a little more, spread the dates out over a month.

Keeping up with the Dow Jones

Spice up your weekend with a few of life's big luxuries with a little price tag.

YOU WILL NEED:

- A luxurious hotel (you don't have to own it, but it has to be nearby)
- A smart suit (for guys) and gorgeous dress (for girls)
- Swimming attire (if applicable)

WHAT TO DO:

We've established you're poor, and you like to get up to kinkiness with each other. So why not take a tip from how the other half live, get dressed up, and head to the most opulent hotel in town. Breeze through the doors like you're guests, and spend the day enjoying the lavish surroundings. You will have to spend a bit of cash, but not as much as you would if you were staying there. Try out some of the following flirty fun before you head home.

- Breakfast on the veranda: some hotels have a continental, serve-yourself breakfast that doesn't require a room number, otherwise shell out for a couple of coffees and a muffin.

- Laze in the lounge: read the complimentary newspapers, enjoy the soothing background music, and cuddle up together on the giant sofas of the hotel's lounge or lobby.

- Hide and peek: hotels are big and there are many places to fool around without getting caught.

- Last orders: don't eat dinner, but sit at the bar and eat cocktail olives, onions, and peanuts, while getting drunk. Flirt the rest of the night away and then head back to your place for the kind of dirty sex people usually reserve for hotel rooms.

SEXONOMIC BONUS:

You hardly need a bonus – you just spent the day hanging out with the 1 per cent for a fraction of the price, but if you keep costs down, be sure to check out the hotel's spa and take a dip in the pool (for a fee), get a massage (for a bigger fee) or snog in the sauna.

FRUGAL RATING:

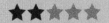

It's going to cost you a bit to pay for all those drinks, snacks and tips, but you'll check out feeling like you checked in, without the hotel bill to match.

Business Sexpenses

Transform your bedroom into a businessman's boudoir for a night of passion (at the company's expense).

No need to steal from the office for this one, but make sure you head home 'with the flu' to get a few extra paid hours out of work to pull off this stunt. Completely clear your bedroom of all personal items, clothes, pictures, etc. Strip down the bed and put on your best sheets, layer up loads of cushions, and put a few mint chocolates on the pillow. Give the room a thorough clean and spray some air freshener for that business hotel effect. If you have a mini fridge, stock it with some little bottles of booze, peanuts, and water, and if there's time give your bathroom the hotel treatment too, remember to fold the toilet paper to a professional peak. Pack a weekend bag with your clothes and toiletries, and do the same for your partner. When they get home, show them into their hotel suite and make the most of being 'away on business' by bonking like crazy on the hotel's beautifully made bed!

PARK AND RIDE IT

Your love wagon might be an obvious place to get
down and dirty in when you fancy a break from the
bed, but it's not necessarily the cheapest way to get
from A to B. Try out some of these more economical
solutions for getting around while getting down and
turn commutes and day trips into travelling turn-ons.

Rate of Return Journey

Convert your commute from a boring journey to an erotic role-play adventure.

YOU WILL NEED:

- A train-journey commute

WHAT TO DO:

Plan with your partner which day of the week you're going to try this out. Rather than meet at the station to catch the train home as usual (or instead of driving your cars to work), board the train alone and find a seat in a quiet carriage. Your partner has to locate you on the train and ask if a seat near to you (preferably next to you) is taken and then sit in it. From this point, you are strangers to each other. You can engage each other in conversation, but only to the point that it seems believable to those around you that you have just met. By the end of the journey, your partner has to try to ask for your number (or vice versa). If they've turned you on enough with their antics to make you want to jump them as soon as you disembark, then give them your details, if not politely refuse and make your way off the train alone, only to meet them in the car park and laugh about your journey. The strangers role-play will get you both hot and bothered that you can't just touch/kiss each other, and the watchful eyes of other commuters will help you stay in character all the way to your stop.

SEXONOMIC BONUS:

Once you've mastered this role-playing ruse, and you almost believe that you've run into a sexy stranger yourself, take this treat to the next level, with a first-class carriage upgrade where there'll be no one around to hear you squeal with delight.

FRUGAL RATING:

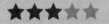

Depending on your commute, and whether you normally drive to work together, catching the train might be more costly than taking your car. But you'll be saving money on parking, can get more work done on the train, and can feel good about doing the green thing. Plus, it's so much easier to flirt when you're not concentrating on the traffic.

Trade Cycle Turn-On

**Get the most out of going to work with a
workout and an eyeful of hot buns.**

YOU WILL NEED:

- A bicycle
- Tight cycling shorts or a more flattering equivalent
- A horn/bicycle bell

WHAT TO DO:

Driving to work is a boring hell of traffic, traffic and more
traffic. If you and your partner need a kick-start in the morning
that also conveniently gets you to the office without all the
hold-ups, then you should try this activity on for size. Squeeze
your peachy behinds into cycling shorts and ride your bikes to
work instead. Your heart will be racing, the wind will be flying
through your hair (unless the law stipulates that you must wear
a helmet), and you'll arrive at work feeling refreshed and ready
for the day. Oh, and let's not forget you get to stare at each

other's backsides all the way there. Honk your bike horn or ring your bell to show your appreciation for your partner's behind throughout the journey. The cycle home is even more fun. Meet up, and make your way back together (take a more scenic route because you're not in any hurry), catch up on each other's days as you go and have a sneaky kiss every time you stop at traffic lights. When you arrive home all hot and sweaty strip off and jump in the shower together – you'll feel so energised that that quick rinse will soon turn into a long sexy soak.

SEXONOMIC BONUS:

Cycling isn't just a great way to get to work – make the most of your new found peddle power by getting on your bike and out of town at the weekend. Stop off at a local pub by a cycle path for refreshments.

FRUGAL RATING:

Unless you have to shell out for new cycling gear, this is a muscle toning money-saver that will get you to work, give you the ass you want, and the ass you want to look at.

Capital Coach Strip

Soak up the romantic city sights without spending like royalty.

YOU WILL NEED:

- A discount coach fare for you and your partner to a big city
- Change for bus fares
- A tourist map
- A picnic

WHAT TO DO:

Normally, we want to get to places as quickly and efficiently as possible. But on a rainy day, there's nothing more enjoyably than canoodling with your partner on a long coach trip to the capital (or any other city you prefer). If you book far enough in advance, and don't care about the time you go, then you can get ridiculously cheap fares to travel between some of the largest cities in the country. Stock up on snacks, pack a picnic for your lunch and spend a few hours relaxing together at the back of the bus. If it's quiet, get away with some subtle sexual behaviour and if you're not shy, unbutton, unzip and discreetly undress a little for your partner. As the bus rumbles along make sure you get some of those good vibrations. When you arrive at your destination, be sure to explore the sights – don't get a tour bus, but hop on a normal city bus for a fraction of the cost and jump off when you see something worth a closer look. When you're done, climb aboard for your return coach trip making sure you rub yourself seductively along the way – you'll be gagging for it by the time you get home.

SEXONOMIC BONUS:

Sure, you're not going to be able to get much sexy time on a coach with a load of grannies, so if you've been saving for a while, treat yourselves to a night at a budget hotel, and head there to heat things up as soon as you arrive.

FRUGAL RATING:

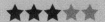

Travelling for fun is not an essential way to spend your pennies, but you'll save a fortune on petrol and parking if you do fancy a city day-trip, and you'll spend less time yelling at each other about whose fault it was that you took that left and more time sucking face.

Credit Car Clean-Up

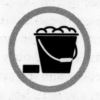

Keep your car clean and your mind filthy.

YOU WILL NEED:

- A car
- Your sexiest/most-revealing swimwear: bikinis for girls and Speedos for guys
- A bucket filled with hot, soapy water
- A hose pipe (optional)
- A sponge

WHAT TO DO:

There's a reason car washes in movies always feature scantily clad girls with hose pipes: it's hot! If you don't have a car, borrow one from a friend and tell them you'll return it all clean (you could even charge them for the privilege and be quids in). Get dressed up in your most revealing swimwear (this goes for both guys and girls) and tell your partner to mow the lawn, or relax in the garden (in full-view of where the car's parked). Fill a bucket with hot, soapy water and head out to start 'cleaning' the car. Take your time pouring the hot water onto the car and rubbing in the soap suds with the sponge; bending, stretching and pushing your body against the car to make sure you get all wet and soapy too. Use your assets to your advantage – girls, push your breasts against the windshield, and guys flex those moist, soapy muscles. Hose the car down with the same sexually consumed expression on your face, and if it's hot, rinse yourself with the cool water too. Try to remain oblivious to your partner, whose jaw will be somewhere on the floor. Head in to get out of your wet gear and they'll be sure to follow, jaw and all, ready to have their way with you the way you had yours with the car (that's if they don't get to you sooner in full view of the neighbours!).

SEXONOMIC BONUS:

Hit the back of the net with this one, and treat yourselves to an automated car wash next time round. Make the most of your time trapped in your vehicle, by fondling, fumbling, and frisking each other as the rollers swish over the windscreen.

FRUGAL RATING:

There's no point paying for a professional cleaning service when you can do it yourself and get done by your lover in the process. Good job!

QUICK WIN TO GET IT IN

Green Shoots and Scores

These boots were made for walking... Take your boots and your booty for a fieldy fun time.

Your frugal rating is going to go through the roof every time you leave the car at home and choose to walk somewhere instead. Walking alone is rarely sexy but it is worth making the effort. The trick is to set off for the shops but make for the countryside and find a field with tall grass – the taller the better. Get down and dirty in the soil and rip off your togs with gusto. Straddle each other and roll around like wild animals until you both look like you walked into a casting for cavemen, rather than to the nearest supermarket. Don't forget to complete whatever car-replacing chore you set out to do while you're grinning from ear to ear. Next time the word 'walk' is mentioned you will hardly be able to contain yourselves.

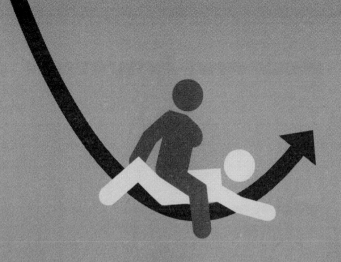

PRIVATE-PART INVESTORS

Whether you've lost your job, hate your job, or can't get a job, the recession has a horrible tendency to make singletons feel even more single. With no money to spend on partying with friends, travelling to exotic locations to meet tanned strangers, and even more hours spent working overtime in the sex-free zone of your office cubicle, it's likely your genitals are feeling as depressed as you are. A lot of the activities in this book can be carried out with new sexual partners or one night stands, but the next few are specifically targeted towards those looking to get some pussy or penis pampering without having to spend your pennies.

Risk and Reward

**A night at the casino will soon become
a naughty night to remember.**

YOU WILL NEED:

• Your hottest outfit

• A fun and flirty girlfriend or wingman to come along with you

WHAT TO DO:

You might think a casino is the worst place to have a good
time when the economy is down, but the rich are always
getting richer, so it's about time you got your fair share of
the winnings. Enjoy your own perfectly innocent, yet utterly
indecent proposal – put on your hottest attire, call your
best friend (or go alone if you're up for it), and head to an
upscale casino. Sit at the bar or in the lounge with a drink
and enjoy yourself. You'll be looking so hot and mysterious
that you're sure to be approached by men with money or
rich divorcees, and from that point onwards you can flirt
the night away without spending a thing. Let them buy you

drinks, gamble their chips, blow on their dice, and then see where the night takes you. A great way to get hot singletons going, is to bet more than money on each roll of the dice or hand of cards, e.g. 'If it's black, I'll go down on you in the toilets.' Those who win big on the table, want to score big in the bedroom too, so you might be up for the wildest night of your life. And screw it, if no proposals take your fancy, call it a night, drunk-dial your bonk buddy, or head home for some alone time, knowing that you got your kicks for free.

SEXONOMIC BONUS:

If you and your friend both find a fun playmate at the casino, take the party back to someone's house for a few rounds of strip poker before bed.

FRUGAL RATING:

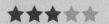

While some might say it's immoral to allow perfect strangers to spend their money on you without offering them something in return, a bit of harmless flirting is all you're really 'rogue' trading here. If you show your willing host a good time in the casino, there's no need to take it any further, unless you just can't resist.

Impressive Figures

Make an exhibition of yourself at the gym to heat up and hook up.

YOU WILL NEED:

- A sexy workout outfit
- A gym class that lets you show off your best moves: weight-lifting, boxing class, street dance, etc.

WHAT TO DO:

Nightclubs are full of sweat, full of competition, and full of idiots. A great place to show off your moves and your body in an unthreatening, booze-free and friendly environment is in a gym. Pick up a free one-week pass to a fancy club or head to your local leisure centre and choose a class that attracts people you're interested in and allows you to flex your muscles the way you do best. This might be a weight-training or boxing class or a hip-hop or pole-dancing workout. Put your all into the exercise routine so all eyes are secretly on you, whether they're the jealous looks of other people working out with you or the double-takes from those peering through the glass. Move it like you're working the bar or on the dancefloor and your figure is sure to become the centre of attention in under an hour. Pull this off and you'll be picking up on your way to the changing room before you've even showered. No door charge, no hangover, and a pool of hotties just waiting to wipe the sweat from your brow after a different kind of workout.

SEXONOMIC BONUS:

Head to the juice bar and get to know your new gym buddy. If you're feeling their flow make sure you have reserves of energy because they're going to want to work your body in ways that guarantee you're going to need a cool-down stretch afterwards.

FRUGAL RATING:

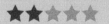

Gym memberships don't come cheap, so if the local leisure centre doesn't appeal make sure you make an impression during your one-week trial, join a running group or start working out in the park to get your super body noticed.

Between the Balance Sheets

Cut down on the costs of the single life by treating yourself to a dirty day in bed.

YOU WILL NEED:

- Your favourite vibrator (have a few toys on standby though), vibrating cock ring or trusty hand
- Spare batteries (if required)
- Inspirational materials (erotic novels, porn movies, magazines, etc.)
- Your finest, freshly washed sheets (optional)

WHAT TO DO:

After a whole week of slugging through hell at work, it's no wonder you want to blow off steam, head to a bar, go out to eat, and treat yourself to some new things at the weekend, but right now, that's money you don't have. Don't punish yourself with solitary confinement, but treat yourself to a whole day of pleasure that hardly requires you to leave your bed. Tell all your friends the day before that you're feeling ill and that you're spending Saturday in bed. This will only be a half-lie. Make sure your freshest, softest sheets are on the bed the night before (if the scent of clean bedding gets you going) and have a lazy morning waking up slowly. When you feel like having some fun, get out your favourite sex toys and trusty turn-ons and have the ultimate masturbation session. After each orgasm, give yourself a few minutes to recover and then get right back into the fun, until your hands are aching or the batteries in your favourite toys have fizzled out. If you're feeling extra frugal, only use your hands, dildos, and other sexy props that don't use batteries to keep yourself entertained. Food and fluid breaks are advised.

SEXONOMIC BONUS:

After you think you couldn't come any more, run yourself a deep, hot bath with salts or bubbles and soak in the tub – you'll be touching yourself in no time.

FRUGAL RATING:

Taking the time to enjoy your body is frugal thinking at its best. No costs are involved and afterwards you're going to feel so relaxed, rewarded and ready for the rest of the week.

QUICK WIN TO GET IT IN

Sex-Efficiency

Play the sex stock market like a pro and end up with the highest return and the most pleasure.

As a working person, you don't have time to get it in as and when you please. You've got food to buy, a house to clean, friends to hang out with... Heading to bars and nightclubs, and just waiting around to be propositioned is costly and an inefficient use of your time. Remember, time is money. Maximise your chance for sex, and increase the return you're getting from your investment by using every opportunity as a chance to hook up. When you're doing the food shopping, make sexy comments about the fresh produce to the cute assistant stocking the bananas, when you're in transit, start up a witty conversation with the bulging biceps or fabulous breasts reading the newspaper. When you're getting your workout, make eyes at the person on the adjacent treadmill. Stop wasting money and time and inject a little sex-efficiency into your pick-up routine.

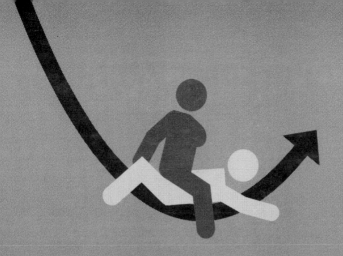

STRIPPED-DOWN SHAREHOLDERS

With friends like these, who needs money? While it's great to have sex on tap with a partner in tow, some things are much more fun when you're hanging with your friends, flirting with your friends, and getting off with your friends. Friends are a cost-free way to keep yourself entertained during the recession – and if you're not feeling like frolicking with any of your nearest and dearest, make sure they get their sexy single mates involved in the following activities so you can improve your shagging stats without blowing your budget (or someone else's partner).

Porkulus Party

Turn a back garden BBQ into a meaty mix of sexy fun for all!

YOU WILL NEED:

- A barbeque
- Hotdog buns
- A little booze never hurts

WHAT TO DO:

If you're sick and tired of hanging out with just your mates, organise a real meaty fest to bring the breasts, thighs and rump steaks right to your door. Throw a huge BBQ, and invite all your friends and their friends. Be sure to emphasise that this is a meaty event, and request that everyone bring some tasty meat to the party (this applies to the food they bring and the fact they must be accompanied by a single friend!). All you need to do is source a cheap bulk supply of burger and hotdog buns and then watch the meat strut in through the door. Keep guests entertained and at the party as long as possible with a hot tub (if you have one!) and other playthings (footballs, basketballs, rugby balls, Frisbees, etc.) that involve everyone playing, touching and getting closer. Keep the booze flowing and your back garden will soon be the perfect place to hook up – all the men will be vibeing off the caveman atmosphere, and all the girls will be giddy from the sun and endless sipping. Sooner or later everyone's going to want to get their hands on some real meat.

SEXONOMIC BONUS:

If you hook up at your party, chances are you'll be the last two left standing. Enjoy a post-coital platter of cold sausages and cheese burgers, or head out for a salad and a smoothie to get refreshed after your extreme meat-fest.

FRUGAL RATING:

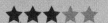

Sure, you have to supply some bread and a little alcohol, but you'll have an entire meat buffet to choose from (and that's not to mention the food!).

Oh, David Camera-On!

**No money in the kitty for the latest porn flick?
Make your own!**

YOU WILL NEED:

- A camera (phone or digital will do, but roll
  out the pro-equipment if you have it!)
- A shooting location
- Props

WHAT TO DO:

They say when times are tough, friends come together and
I couldn't agree more – especially about the coming part.
Don't waste your cash on cheap skin flicks or disappointing
downloads – invite your mates over for a few drinks and
once the ice is broken, assign roles to the sexy girls and
guys you know (make sure you're in the movie too!). Get
everyone to act out a load of hilarious and horny moments
that would build up to a full-on filthy porn scene. They

probably won't want to take the fun too far, but the flirty fiction you create is likely to get any funemployed friend hot and bothered. Capture the whole show on camera (edit it and add in music, if you're that way inclined) and then screen the film for the group at the end of the night.

SEXONOMIC BONUS:

Dash out for a few extra bottles of cheap wine and microwave some popcorn to celebrate your sexy debuts, and see where the evening goes.

FRUGAL RATING:

Cheaper than a night out of drinking, a little pricier than downloading a movie from your favourite porn site. Either way, it's definitely more fun and a lot more likely to lead to hilarious, out-of-hand, drunken and dirty behaviour between your friends. Yay!

Naughty NASDAQ!

An efficient way to rate the singles you know, the singles you don't, and the singles you want to know more intimately.

YOU WILL NEED:

- A social networking site or online dating account
- A computer
- Some paper and pens
- Your most trusted allies

WHAT TO DO:

Time is money people and none of us are getting any younger. If you wanted to know what stock to invest in, you'd ask a broker, so it makes perfect sense that you get together with your mates and judge the evidence to determine who is worthy of each other's charms. Pull up each other's potential investments' profiles on social networking sites or on the dating network pages that they've approached you on. Make sure everyone has a pen and paper to write down their scores. Give each candidate a score out of 10 on the following categories.

Looking pretty – How hot do you think they are?

Making money – Does it appear that they're going to cripple your friend's financial situation or save it? Check their job credentials.

Talking shit – How much do you think your friend and the candidate will have to talk about?

Anyone who scores 22/30 or higher is worth you or your friend's time – call them up immediately and set up a date. Otherwise, check the stock market in a few weeks and see if anything more appealing takes your fancy.

SEXONOMIC BONUS:

Brokers earn a good living, so it's only fair that your advisors get something in return for their wisdom. Cook your mates a meal or buy everyone a pint at the pub afterwards – if you're all helping each other out, make it a potluck or BBQ – and toast to your future financial (and dating) success!

FRUGAL RATING:

It costs nothing to take the time do a thorough inspection of any investment before you waste time and money going for a drink with it, and your friends will have a good laugh rating your potential partners.

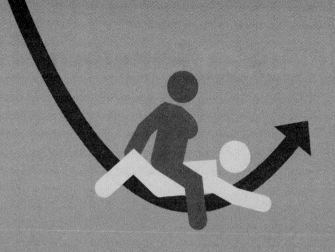

DAY TRADER
TURN-ONS

*We know that just because you're arriving at work early,
staying late, and doing everything within socially acceptable
limits to get your boss to give you a pay rise, it doesn't mean
you can't have a little flirty fun from 9–5. If you have a job,
you're probably trying your damndest to keep it, which
means that you can't afford to flake off for erotic excursions
and sexual 'sick' days. Make the most of all that time you're
spending working your arse off, and make sure your arse is
getting some of the loving it deserves while you're there.*

Elevation Stimulation

What goes up, must be willing to go down there and enjoy some fondling friction.

YOU WILL NEED:

- A tall office building with a lift
- A willing man/woman (either your partner, or someone you're intimately acquainted with)

WHAT TO DO:

Taking the lift in the morning may be the quickest way to get to your desk and earn your crust but it's hardly stimulating. Introduce the rewarding risk of having to give your partner an intimate frisk while you wait to arrive at your floor. When you get into the lift, make sure you're the only people around. Hit the button for your floor (or head to a higher floor if you want to give yourselves more time) and then stick your hand inside their underwear and get to work. If the lift stops at a floor to let someone on, you can decide whether to stop immediately, leaving your partner wanting more, to carry on discreetly (which could be tricky), or to press your backside into your partner's crotch to keep them stimulated until you're left alone again. If you don't work in the same office as your partner, you could try this out when you visit other people's offices – lawyers, dentists, etc. – otherwise try to recreate a similar high-risk hand-job scenario in other situations, like in taxis or at a family gathering.

SEXONOMIC BONUS:

It's unlikely you're going to have time to get your partner off completely in a short elevator ride (unless you have super sexy skills), so meet them on your break somewhere private to finish the job and eat your lunch to celebrate.

FRUGAL RATING:

You're definitely not going to save much money out of this one, but it will get your engines going first thing, and your partner will definitely work harder in the morning knowing what to expect at lunchtime.

Callateral Dirty Damage

Pick up line one and dial your date for a working day phone sex workout.

YOU WILL NEED:

- An office crush (optional)
- A phone at your desk
- An internal number

WHAT TO DO:

Save money on sending flirty texts and stop wasting time with indirect emails. The best way to get your pulse racing is to pick up the phone and tell your partner, lover or office crush exactly what you want to do to them and hear them talking about your body like it's an exciting toy they want to play with. If you work at a desk or in a cubicle, part of the thrill comes from wondering if you're being overheard, and having to quickly divert the conversation when someone comes into your office or approaches your desk. Tell your partner to repeat things out loud that you've told them you want them to do to you. This form of phone sex works even better if your partner or lover works in the same building or even in the same open-plan office. If anyone asks, you're not making a personal call; you're simply discussing the latest figures for blah, blah, blah... The perfect cover.

SEXONOMIC BONUS:

Although it's probably frowned upon, there's nothing quite like screwing on your desk, under your desk, or on your boss's desk. You've been working so many late nights that no one will think it's weird that you stay behind to 'finish up'. Have your regular bed-fellow head over to your office for a change of scenery and then screw them until they feel like they spent the whole day working in your office too.

FRUGAL RATING:

Sure, you're not saving much, but you're making the most of the office facilities in a way that is much more pleasurable to you. And you'll certainly never look at your desk the same way again.

Trolley Dolly Discount

Bid farewell to Starbucks and start sexing up tea-break time in your office.

YOU WILL NEED:

(All the following should be provided by the office)
- A trolley or a tray
- Tea/coffee/milk/sugar
- Kettle/coffee machine

Girls you will need:
- Low-cut shirt, skirt, sexy shoes

Boys you will need:
- Tight-fitting shirt unbuttoned at the top
- Fitted trousers that emphasise your package

WHAT TO DO:

Stepping out of the office for a grande double-shot soy vanilla latte is a privilege of the rich. You are not rich, and therefore need to stop spending your 'spare' change on frothy coffees and fragrant herbal teas. Your office has a break room, and in it you will find all the essentials for making perfectly adequate tea and coffee. Inspire everyone to save, by dressing up once a week in your sexy apparel that says, 'I'm not just here for light refreshments.' Your sexy new look is sure to attract the attention of all your prospectively up-for-it co-workers. Do a whip around the office to take everyone's order, make the beverages and then deliver them to your grateful colleagues with a tray. Girls, be sure to bend low and close to your office crush when you hand-deliver their beverage. Guys, be sure to proudly display your own sugar lump to whoever you fancy. You'll be sure to have a number of eligible tea-making assistants when tea-break time comes around next week.

SEXONOMIC BONUS:

Wearing particular sexy or fitted clothes to work (especially if you don't normally) will get you heaps of attention from the hotties in the office.

FRUGAL RATING:

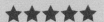

Drinking office supplies, even if it requires standing next to a kettle for a few minutes and a bit of stirring, is going to save you money every single day, and you'll certainly be stirring up the office with your sexy new look and personal service.

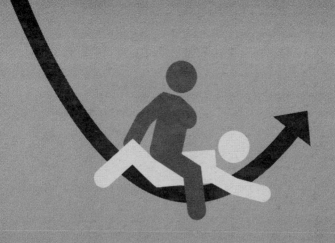

F-ING FRUGAL EXCHANGE

After shagging and saving your way through this book, you should be in better shape financially and sexually. Tally up how many activities you have successfully completed (or at least attempted!) and see where your sexy stock is ranked on the F-ing Frugal Exchange.

1–15: BONER BROKER

If you've only just started, this level of commitment may
be forgiven, but otherwise you really need to get back
on that horse and ride like a slutty cowboy/girl. Work is
stressful, and can get in the way of the giant schlong or
perky breasts your partner's been walking around the house,
so introduce a little fun into the office (DAY TRADER TURN-
ONS), or take a cheap and sexually charged trip (TAKE A
BREAK AND BONK WHILE BEING BROKE) to get your
libido and your budget back on track.

16–30: SOFT INVESTOR

Yes, you're starting to achieve the easiest part of the Recession
Kama Sutra – the sex part – but every time you do an activity
you reward yourself with a costly Sexonomic Bonus, cancelling
out your savings. Sure you might be turned on a lot more,
but focus on activities with the higher Frugal Ratings and
you'll start to see some movement in your bank balance,
as well as your partner's underwear. Make the recession
your bitch and pump up the volume so that your sex life
shoots through the roof right alongside your finances.

31–45: HIGH YIELDER

Things are looking good – you're saving cash and walking around with a giant grin on your face from all the sexual gratification you've been getting. Now it's time to focus on putting those savings to good use and not getting complacent. The sex might be on tap right now, but if you want to see the other side of this recession with savings and a sex life this good, you're going to have to invest in the future. Make sure your partner is offering the same commitment to putting money aside and taking you for the ride of your life and you'll be well on your way to sexy money harmony.

46–60: HOT MONEY MAKER

You are proof that with a little time, a lot of effort, and even more positions than you can count, anyone can fight off the recession with their mind and their sexy parts. You've taken all these activities in your stride, given them a try, and found what works for you. No matter where the economy is headed you know you're getting head, and headed south for some good times. You have money in the bank and you ain't afraid to show it. Oh yeah, you're sexy and you know it!

VERY
NAUGHTY
GAMES

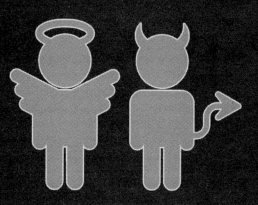

TARA TING

VERY NAUGHTY GAMES

Tara Ting

ISBN: 978-1-84953-113-9

£5.99

Hardback

Hussy Roulette

You Will Need:

- A bottle
- A pair of handcuffs
- A spanking tool
- A bucket of ice cubes

Grown-ups only! This sexy stocking-full of seductive games will get you hot under the collar and ready for cheeky action in no time. From frisky foreplay to duvet dalliances, there's a suggestion here for every occasion, including **Pleasure Hunt**, **Eurovision Strip Contest** and **Snogging For Apples**. So slip into something more comfortable and get in the mood for naughtiness – it's time to play!

Fifty Shades
of *Bliss*

The ultimate guide to
spicing up your sex life

LEXIE SUTTON

FIFTY SHADES OF BLISS

The ultimate guide to spicing up your sex life

Lexie Sutton

ISBN: 978-1-84953-365-2

£6.99

Paperback

Treat yourself and your lover to *Fifty Shades of Bliss*!

If you've been seduced by Christian and Anastasia's erotic adventures in *Fifty Shades of Grey*, this is just the book you need to help you turn your fantasies into reality. With fifty raunchy chapters leading you from 'vanilla' sex all the way to sinful BDSM delights, this handy no-holds-barred guide is packed with delicious hints, tips and eye-opening ideas for exploring naughty and thrilling new games together.

Playful and practical, and covering everything from stripping to submission, this sweet treat of a book will lead you and your partner to blissful new heights.

If you're interested in finding out more about
our humour books, follow us on Twitter:
@SummersdaleLOL

www.summersdale.com